I0765859

Essential Oils for Dandruff

Essential Oil Recipes for
Dandruff
for Diffusers, Roller Bottles,
Inhalers & more.

Rica V. Gadi

Copyright © 2019 by The Oil Natural Empress

All rights reserved. This book or any portion thereof may not be reproduced or used in any manner whatsoever without the express written permission of the publisher except for the use of brief quotations in a book review.

Printed in the United States of America

First Printing, 2019

ISBN: 9781690019305

http://eorecipes.net

DISCLAIMER: This document is a compilation of recipes used successfully by EO enthusiasts who use only high-quality, therapeutic-grade essential oils as determined by many factors including growth, growth location, harvesting process, distillation method used, etc. Please be advised that not all essential oils are created equally, and not all essential oils are suitable for topical use or ingestion. Please do your research before choosing the brand(s) of essential oils you decide to use as well as the supplies you use. Always follow label directions on the essential oil bottles.

All the recipes in this book have been inspired by essential oil believers. However, we are not medical practitioners and do not diagnose, treat or prescribe treatment for any health condition or disease. Just a precaution, before using any alternative medicine, natural supplements, or vitamins, you should always discuss the products you are using or intend to use with your doctor, especially if you are pregnant, trying to get pregnant or nursing.

All information contained within this book is for reference purposes only, and is not intended to substitute for advice given by a pharmacist, physician or other licensed health-care professional. As such, the author is not responsible for any loss, claim or damage arising from the use of the essential oil recipes contained herein.

This book is dedicated to all the strong people who are taking responsibility for your own well being and doing something to be better.

All my heartfelt gratitude to the following people: my mom Ruby Jane, you have made me everything I am today; my dad Nestor-- my eternal, my angel, and the source of my perseverance; Mommyling, my spiritual guide ; Ria & Joe, the true witnesses of my transformation and my foundation pillars; Ellie Jane, the sparkle of our eyes;

Juan, thanks for always encouraging me to push harder - you are my ONE; Rocco & Radha, my reason for everything.

The Love of my family and friends is the fountain of inspiration that never runs dry. Thank you for constantly inspiring me, motivating me, and loving me unconditionally.

This book will never be complete without the help of my trusted and talented friends the #NOWsuperstars and my #oilbularya friends

Blending Essential Oils to use for a very specific reason has become very popular in recent years. There are several reasons why this is so. Blending EOs is basically about inhaling - as it has been proven that aromas have the ability to trigger feelings, emotions and personal memories.

With this in mind, it is obvious that everyone is unique when it comes to what triggers your senses. It all boils down to personal preference for the aroma to trigger what you want to unleash. Everyone is different and we all connect to the aroma differently, so what might work for one might not work for another person.

Of course, we also want the blend we personalize to be therapeutic. This is the best reason why to blend essential oils. We want the blend we create to help us with a very specific emotion or physical conditions. As much as smelling good is important in a blend, it is more important that we blend oils that are not only pleasing to the smell but also produces the therapeutic effect we are after.

Then you have to think about contraindications. Making sure the blend you create is safe to use.

I suggest that before blending, find out if the oils you are using are safe for a condition you may have, for example, if you are pregnant, or have specific allergies. Consult your physician prior to moving forward.

The recipes I have in this book is a compilation of what has proven to work and favored by hundreds of EO enthusiasts. It takes out the guesswork to get you started.

Again, we urge you to read the recipes and make sure that this is safe for you to try.

The book is very specific to a physical and emotional condition. There are several recipes here because you might want to rotate and you may like one and not the other. There are also a variety of applications. Some of us prefer to diffuse, some to make roller bottles, and others to create inhalers and sprays.

I hope you enjoy this compilation, feel free to use the notes section and jot down your fave blends. There is a wonderful world of EO blending - this is just the beginning.

Rica

A minor but very common skin condition that many people experience is called dandruff. This is a skin condition that affects our scalp. It causes itchiness, dryness and excess skin flakes on the scalp. This can be embarrassing or seen as an unhygienic thing to have. When somebody has dandruff, it is often seen as neglect on a proper hair care routine. There are plenty of other causes of dandruff and it is important to know so we can be aware of the changes we need to do in order to avoid it. Dandruff is usually caused by a yeast or fungal infection that spread in the scalp. This can be particularly difficult to treat when the scalp is sensitive or has open wounds and other problems. Over-washing or under-washing of the hair can also be a cause of dandruff as it affects the oiliness and dryness of the scalp. Environmental factors such as dust, dirt, and moisture are also some conditions that may cause the build-up of dandruff.

Dandruff is generally not a dangerous condition to have, although it may be very uncomfortable. There are plenty of effective daily routines to do to help reduce or cure dandruff without the need to go to the doctor. Basic hygiene such as washing your hair with the right products can cure dandruff easily. Taking good care of your health by eating the right kinds of food and drinking lots of water is another natural way to avoid dandruff because the food and drinks we take in affect the reactions that happen in our skin and body. For a faster and more direct way to help treat dandruff, some people use essential oils. It does not instantly cure dandruff but it is a great alternative to help treat and soothe it. It is one of the best natural home remedies that can be prepared in a matter of minutes.

Some of the best essential oils to use to get rid of dandruff on the scalp are tea tree oil, lavender oil, peppermint oil, and patchouli oil. Tea tree oil is known for its antiseptic properties that disinfect and help kill germs and bacteria. A lot of people also use this to treat acne. It has soothing properties that cool the scalp and helps alleviate itchiness and inflammation. Lavender oil is also quite similar but it focuses more on anti-fungal properties. Dandruff is usually caused by yeasts and this is a fungal infection that is properly treated by lavender oil. Peppermint oil, on the other hand, can help treat dandruff by providing a cooling sensation to the scalp and help reduce redness and itchiness as well.

Table of Contents

Essential Oils for Dandruff

If you're the victim of a flaky scalp, you know that struggle is real. While flakes of any sort can arise, it's actually an excess of oil that causes true dandruff. The most common thing to do if you're in any kind of flake predicament is swing by your local drugstore and pick up a bottle of dandruff shampoo, which tends to contain the active ingredients known as selenium sulfide or zinc pyrithione. However, if dandruff shampoos aren't for you, or you want to go a more natural route, essential oils could be worth a try.

1. Chamomile Essential Oil

Chamomile essential oil is another useful natural hair treatment. Whether your hair is excessively oily or excessively dry, chamomile essential oils help balance out the conditions of the hair. Chamomile essential oil also effectively reduces inflammation and soothe the itchiness that typically accompanies dandruff.

Chamomile essential oil can even be used to lighten the tones of the hair when mixed with baking soda and applied topically. Hair treated with chamomile oil is shinier and softer than hair treated with synthetic.

2. Lavender Essential Oil

Clinical studies have just started to examine the effects of lavender essential oil on hair health. Lavender essential oil is a potent antibacterial and antifungal. If dandruff has resulted in itchiness or irritation, especially when caused by stress, lavender essential oils soothe the skin and the mind.

Lavender essential oils had a significant effect on the health of the skin's thermal layer and the depth of hair follicles. It was even found to increase the number of follicles in female test subjects, possibly due to its hormone-balancing effects.

3. Frankincense Essential Oil

If you're not dealing with dandruff, but instead a dry scalp, this EO might be your ticket. "Applying frankincense regularly will regulate the scalp's moisture," says Brown. She recommends applying frankincense oil post hair wash so your scalp is squeaky clean, which will help the oils absorb into your skin. Start with one drop of frankincense to four ounces of castor oil and then adjust, depending on your needs. Put on a shower cap for 15 minutes and shampoo again. Repeat as often as needed to keep the flakes under control.

4. Cedarwood Oil

Cedarwood essential oil is a great treat after a long stressful day. By improving blood flow through the scalp, this essential oil improves the health of your hair from the roots. Cedarwood essential oil also has well-established antifungal properties.

Scottish scientists set out to test the properties of cedarwood essential oil, used in combination with other essential oils, to remedy alopecia—hair loss on the scalp. The results showed a 44 percent improvement in comparison to control groups results. Furthermore, cedarwood essential oils are an effective remedy for lice, fleas, and ticks.

5. Rosemary Oil

Rosemary essential oil is among the most versatile of natural hair treatments. Studies have found that rosemary essential oil can boost the rate of cellular metabolism, resulting in hair growth and restoration of the scalp and follicles.

6. Tea Tree Essential Oil

Tea tree essential oil contains powerful antiseptic, antimicrobial and antibacterial properties that kills bacteria, yeast and germs that accumulate on the scalp and cause dandruff. It provides a soothing and cooling sensation when applied to an itchy & inflamed scalp caused by dandruff.

Although tea tree essential oil can be used neat on the skin, some people, especially those with sensitive skin can experience burning sensations. Therefore, please ensure to mix it with a carrier oil like jojoba, coconut or olive oil to stay on the safe side.

7. Thyme Essential Oil

Containing strong antifungal & antiseptic properties, thyme essential oil staves off any germs & fungi that causes dandruff and scalp infections. Thyme essential oil also invigorates the scalp thereby stimulating circulation in the scalp, which helps keep the scalp healthy and dandruff-free.

There are many different ways to enjoy the benefits of essential oils for the hair. Shampoos, hair masks, and direct topical application with carrier oils are all great options. Remember that a small amount goes a long way and consistency always brings out the best results. Try using one or a mix of the essential oils mentioned for a safe, natural dandruff remedy.

The Blending Process

These EOs are categorized by aromas, and EOs from the same group usually blend fantastically together.

- Floral – Lavender, Geranium, Jasmine
- Woodsy – Pine, Cedarwood
- Earthy – Vetiver, Patchouli
- Herbaceous – Marjoram, Rosemary, Basil
- Minty – Peppermint, Spearmint, Wintergreen
- Medicinal – Eucalyptus, Frankincense, Melaleuca
- Spicy – Pepper, Clove, Cinnamon
- Oriental – Ginger, Patchouli
- Citrus – Wild Orange, Lemon, Lime

Select oils that will give you the health benefits you are looking to remedy. For increased energy choose: Grapefruit, Lemon, Orange, or Citrus. For Calming and Relaxation choose: Lavender, Cedarwood, or Chamomile. You are encouraged to experiment and play with your oils to see which blends work for you.

TIPS:

- Combine Floral EOs with Woodsy, Spicy and Citrus aromas
- Minty EOs with Woodsy, Earthy, Herbaceous and Citrus aromas
- Earthy EOs with Woodsy and Minty aromas
- Citrus EOs with Floral, Woodsy, Minty, Spicy and Oriental aromas

Essential Oils Substitution List

Sometimes we want to blend oils but we just don't have all the oils as stated in a recipe. I've created an easy to use guide for substitution.

Name of Oil	SUB 1	SUB 2	SUB 3
Arborvitae	Melissa	Cedarwood	Patchouli
Basil	Massage Blend	Marjoram	Thyme
Bergamot	Grapefruit	Lime	
Birch	Wintergreen	Cypress	
Black Pepper	Copaiba	Juniper Berry	Clove
Blue Tansy	Roman Chamomile		
Cardamom	Lavender	Clary Sage	Roman Chamomile
Cassia	Cinnamon		
Cedarwood	Arborvitae	Patchouli	Vetiver
Cellular Blend	Frankincense	Thyme	Clove
Cilantro	Coriander	Cardamom	Black Pepper
Cinnamon	Cassia		
Clary Sage	Ylang Ylang		
Clove	Cassia	Cinnamon	
Copaiba	Thyme	Oregano	Clove
Coriander	Lavender	Juniper Berry	Cardamom

Cypress	Douglas Fir	Massage Blend	Copaiba
Detoxification Blend	Geranium	Copaiba	Rosemary
Digestive Blend	Fennel	Peppermint	Ginger
Dill	Bergamot	Lemon	Wild Orange
Douglas Fir	Siberian Fir	Cypress	
Eucalyptus	Respiratory Blend	Melaleuca	Melissa
Frankincense	Cedarwood		
Geranium	Copaiba	Rose	
Ginger	Digestive Blend	Fennel	Geranium
Grapefruit	Bergamot	Lemon	Wild Orange
Helichrysum	Myrrh		
Jasmine	Roman Chamomile	Rose	Ylang Ylang
Juniper Berry	Coriander		
Lavender	Petitgrain	Roman Chamomile	Coriander
Lemon	Wild Orange	Lime	Grapefruit
Lemongrass	Helichrysum	Cilantro	
Marjoram	Basil	Cypress	
Melaleuca	Neroli	Rosemary	Eucalyptus
Melissa	Black Pepper	Eucalyptus	

Metabolic Blend	Ginger	Peppermint	Cinnamon
Myrrh	Sandalwood	Spikenard	
Neroli	Rosemary	Melissa	Melaleuca
Oregano	Thyme	Basil	Copaiba
Patchouli	Vetiver	Focus Blend	Cedarwood
Peppermint	Spearmint		
Petitgrain	Lavender	Wild Orange	Bergamot
Protective Blend	Cinnamon	Clove	Copaiba
Renewing Blend	Bergamot	Juniper Berry	Myrrh
Respiratory Blend	Eucalyptus	Rosemary	Melaleuca
Roman Chamomile	Blue Tansy	Lavender	Focus Blend
Rose	Geranium	Jasmine	Ylang Ylang
Rosemary	Melaleuca	Neroli	Eucalyptus
SandalWood	Cedarwood	Spikenard	Myrrh
Siberian Fir	Douglas Fir	White Fir	Cedarwood
Soothing Blend	Helichrysum	Peppermint	Wintergreen
Spearmint	Peppermint	Reassuring Blend	
Spikenard	Myrrh	Vetiver	Patchouli
Thyme	Oregano	Copaiba	Clove

Vetiver	Patchouli	Spikenard	Cedarwood
White Fir	Siberian Fir	Douglas Fir	
Wild Orange	Tangerine	Lemon	Grapefruit
Wintergreen	Birch	Siberian Fir	
Ylang Ylang	Jasmine	Lavender	

Diffuse

Diffusing Essential Oils is the safest method to enjoy Essential Oils without the risk of an allergic reaction.

Diffusing Essential Oils
Some Tidbits You Need To Know

Our sense of smell is one of our most powerful senses, and as you have noticed in your own experience, some scents affect you more positively in your minds than others. The body contains over 1,000 receptors for smell—way more receptors than for any of our other senses.

Diffusion Essential Oils means the process vaporizes oils into the air by releasing tiny amounts into the air. Inhalation is totally safe and is super low risk. Chances of any EO rising to dangerous levels while diffusion is slim to none.

Diffusing Essential Oils around newborns, babies, young children, pregnant or nursing women, and pets should be done with caution. Read up on safety.

It is advisable that Diffusing Essential Oils for only about 15-30 minutes at a time to be most effective. NEVER leave your diffuser on overnight. Make sure your diffuser is filled with the right amount of water and you understand the operating directions.

While diffusing essential oils, be sure that your space has great ventilation. Crack a window open if the scent becomes strong.

Never add Carrier Oils to your diffuser. This may cause your diffuser to malfunction. Clean your diffuser at least 3 times a week with warm water and natural soap to ensure the diffuser is well maintained and bacteria and mold does not accumulate.

Diffusing Essential Oils
Basic Guidelines

Just a few things you need to know and prepare before getting started Diffusing Essential Oils.

Things you need:
Ultrasonic Oil Diffuser
Essential Oils
Water

Just follow the number of drops in the recipe, drop on to an oil diffuser and fill the rest with water.

All diffusers are different and will have its own water minimum and maximum level. Read the diffuser instruction before use.

Ideally, it is best to diffuse for 15-30 minutes and turn off the diffuser. The effect should be good for at least 2-3 hours. Turn your diffuser back on after 3 hours to reinforce oil diffusing effects.

It is not advisable to use EO in humidifiers.

These are not made to release EOS

Roll

Essential Oil Roller Bottles is the easiest method to enjoy Essential Oils Anywhere and Whenever.

Blending Essential Oils in a Roller Bottle
Some Tidbits You Need To Know

Essential Oils are usually super concentrated and too hard to measure how much to actually put straight from the bottle.

Roller bottles are a way that you are able to create blends ready to use with the right dilution. It allows your EO to last longer.

It also makes it easier to apply exactly where you want to target without getting it all over the place.

It is handy and easy to carry in your purse, ready to use at any time you want to.

I like to apply EOs at the bottom of the feet for many reasons. Our feet have bigger pores than any other skin in our bodies. This means that they are able to suck in the therapeutic compounds in our blend into the bloodstream faster than any other parts of the body. Imagine comparing a normal straw to an oversized straw and how much more you can suck in with the latter. This is how the soles of our feet are compared to the rest of the skin in our bodies.

The skin on our feet is also less sensitive and is designed to withstand some abuse. The risk of having an irritation from EOS is less likely to happen when applied on the feet.

The feet don't have the glands that act as a barrier. Sebaceous glands are glands in our skin that produce an oily substance called Sebum, for the purpose of lubricating and waterproofing the skin. Since this is oil and if you put oil on top of oil, it can act as a barrier or it may slow down penetration.

The feet and palms of our hands are the only skin that don't have these, so it is ideal to apply Essential Oils to the feet for maximum penetration.

Now, it would be hard to apply oils directly and very messy, right? Roller bottles make it super easy and convenient to roll the EOs at the bottom of our feet.

Carrier Oils Info

Carrier oils are vegetable-based oils with their own healing properties that dilute essential oils used to help carry the EOs into the skin.

Essential oils are highly concentrated and could evaporate very quickly. The carrier oil is mixed with the essential oil so it could penetrate the skin before it actually evaporates. Although EOs are oils, it is actually not that oily. When mixed with a carrier oil, it allows you to have more of the essential oil into your skin without wasting EOS to evaporate, making the healing properties of the EO strong and more effective.

There are also Essential oils that are too strong to apply directly to the skin and may cause damage, so it is important to dilute them with carrier oil.

Never add Carrier Oils to your diffuser. This may cause your diffuser to malfunction. Clean your diffuser at least 3 times a week with warm water and natural soap to ensure the diffuser is well maintained and bacteria and mold does not accumulate.

Carrier Oils

There are a lot of different carrier oils that you can use with EOs to dilute them in a roller bottle.

To name a few :

Almond Oil - moisturizing and stays liquid at room temperature. Do not use it if you are allergic to nuts.

Apricot Kernel Oil - moisturizing and suitable for sensitive skin or kids. It is super gentle on the skin.

Avocado Oil - moisturizing and suitable for sensitive and damaged skin. Perfect for skin problems.Can be mixed with other carrier oils

Castor Oil - with antibacterial, antiviral and antifungal properties, use topically to eliminate pain and relieve skin irritation.

Coconut Oil - its antibacterial, antiviral and antifungal properties it is the best and most versatile for skin care. The skin absorbs this very quickly. It solidifies in room temp and may still have a slight coconut oil aroma in it - but you can get fractionated coconut oil to eliminate the 2 challenges above.

Grapeseed Oil - not just for cooking but also great for topical application on the skin.

Jojoba Oil - one of my faves for skin care blends. This oil is the closest to our natural oil our skin produces so it is absorbed easily without being oily. Also amazing for massage oil blends.

Olive Oil - this is the oil for herb type oils. mostly used for cooking but can also be applied to the skin but would need to be blended with a carrier oil that is mild and absorb well with the skin.

Rosehip Seed Oil - super good for deep moisturizing or skin irritations. This oil has a high content of antioxidants and helps remedy dry, scarred and wounded skin.

Recommended Roller Bottle Dilution Guide

RECOMMENDED ROLL-ON BOTTLE DILUTION AMOUNTS

5 ml (1/6 oz.) Roll-on Bottle = ~100 drops (1tsp.)
10 ml (1/3 oz.) Roll-on Bottle = ~200 drops (2 tsp.)
30 ml. (1 oz.) Roll-on Bottle = ~600 drops (6 tsp.)

Roll-on Size	5 ml	10 ml	30 ml	Add EO drops to roll-on, then fill with carrier oil.	
Essential Oil Drops	1	2	6	1%	Dilution Percentage
	2	4	12	2%	
	3	6	18	3%	
	5	10	30	5%	
	10	20	60	10%	
	20	40	120	20%	
	25	50	150	25%	
	50	100	300	50%	

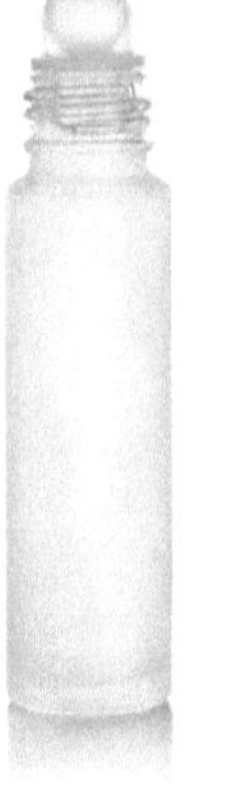
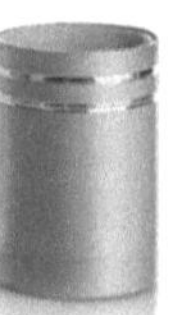

General Guidelines:
Birth to 12 months = .3-.5% dilution
1-5 years = 1.5-3% dilution
6-11 years = 1.5-5% dilution
12-17 years = 1.5-20% dilution
18 years and older = 1.5% dilution-Neat (no dilution)
Elderly or Sensitive Skin = 1-3% dilution
Daily Use = 2-5% dilution
Short Term Use = 10-25% dilution
Local Skin or Systemic Issues = 50% dilution-Neat

These are general guidelines suggestions--not absolute rules--based on traditional aromatheraphy practice.
(Kurt Schnaubelt PhD, Valerie Worwood, Robert Tisserand)

Dilution Basics:

How much you dilute your EO depends on different factors such as weight, sensitivity, health conditions, EOs that are blended in or how long that blend has been used for. There is never an absolute dilution rule, it is you who knows about your level and tolerance. I feel that it is best to start with a higher dilution percentage and increase EO drops over time.

To make sure your EO is safe, make sure that the oils you use are therapeutic grade and do your research on the source and extraction methods used to produce the oils.

Roller Bottle Blending Order

I normally just start with dropping the drops of oil into the **10mL roller bottle**, then adding the carrier oil up until the shoulder of the bottle. Capping the bottle off with the roller and the bottle cap. Instead of shaking the bottle, I like to roll the bottle between my palms first for a minute or 2 for blending, then finishing it off with a few shakes.

NOTE: All recipes in this book are for a 10mL Roller Bottle. If you have a bigger or smaller roller bottle, adjust the number of EO drops based on the size of your bottle.

Inhale

Essential Oil Inhalers are the most convenient way to enjoy Essential Oils Anywhere and Whenever.

Essential Oil Inhalers give you quick and easy access to the vast therapeutic benefits of essential oils.

Blending Essential Oils in an Inhaler
Some Tidbits You Need To Know

EO Inhalers or aroma sticks are compact tubes, with a cotton wick inside and a protective cover, to lock the aroma within.

Your preferred blend of essential oils is absorbed by the cotton wick, and safely enclosed in a tube that fits inside of the cover. The cover is easily removed for access to the tube to breathe in the aroma. Usually lasts about 3 months, depending on the oil blend used.

I absolutely love these because they encourage me to take a moment during super stressful moments, and just breathe.

It is in times of stress when our breathing patterns often change and taking deep breaths promote a feeling of calm and inner peace. Breath work combined with visualization plus a relaxing inhaler, can offer relief to symptoms of stress and help your body to come back to the state of homeostasis.

Aroma Sticks can be carried in your tiny purse, even compact enough to fit in your pocket. You can enjoy your favorite EOs anywhere and you can use them with discretion.

I love diffusing, and do all the time but not everyone in my space may enjoy the scents I enjoy or they may not benefit from the therapeutic benefits of the EOs I am diffusing - so the inhaler is one way to not only enjoy my choice of blends but to keep in personal not affecting everyone else around me.

Inhalers not only benefits me but also keep those around me safe in case the oils I want to blend may pose a risk to those around me who may have a health issue not advised to be exposed to my choice EOs/

When making Aroma Sticks, You may use your chosen EOs at 100% Concentration.

Inhaler Basic Guidelines

Breathe in slow and deep to absorb the EO molecules directly into your olfactory system.

Inhalers are super easy to use. You just remove the cap and inhale from the inhaler tube, count 1 to 5 slowly as you inhale. The EO molecules get drawn into our bloodstream through our nasal cavity and get delivered throughout our entire body.

Simple to use, easy to carry, portable and compact. You never have to be without your favorite blends, ever.

Inhaler Blending Basics

Inhalers are super easy and simple to make.

All you need is an inhaler set which consist of the following:

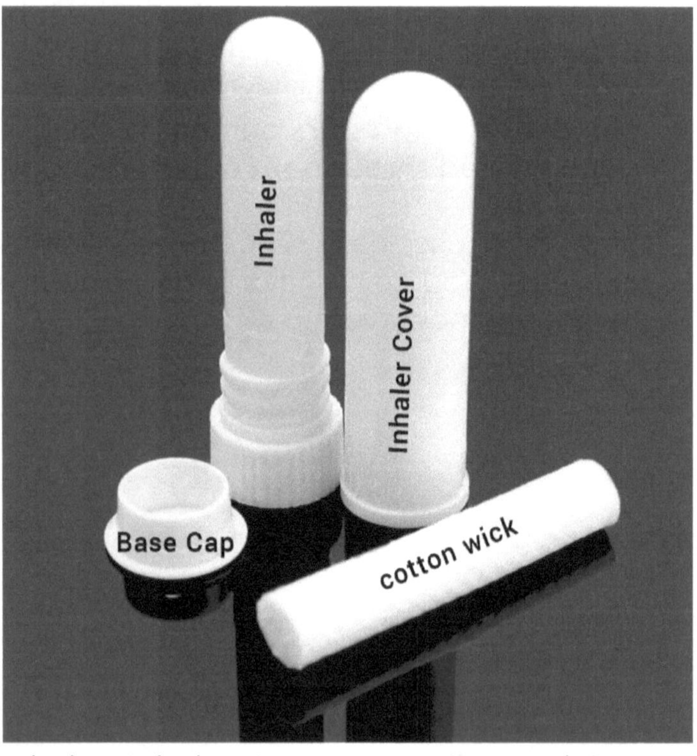

Inhaler, Inhaler Cover, Base Cap and Cotton Wick.

You will need your Essential Oils.

I like to use a pipette for precision and a small petri dish so I can see the oil.

Blending is super easy, just combine the drops and swirl it around in the petri dish and when you are satisfied you can go ahead and drop the cotton wick to absorb all the oil in the dish.

Once the wick is ready you can drop it in the inhaler and cap the bottom with the Base Cap. I usually like to secure the cover with the inhaler so I don't have to do it later.

I usually use 15-20 drops of EO total in a recipe and it can last up to 3 months. Some recipes will need more but on average it is in this range.

EO Recipes for Dandruff

The Best Essential Oils For Hair Growth #1

2 drops thyme essential oil
5 drops lavender essential oil
2 tbsp extra virgin olive oil

Rub the mix into the scalp and let it rest for
20 minutes.

The Best Essential Oils For Hair Growth #2

4 drops helichrysum essential oil
4 drops rosemary essential oil
5 drops lavender essential oil

Rub the mix into the scalp and let it rest for
1-2 hours.

Diy Deep Moisturizing Dry Scalp Treatments #1

4 drops lemon
2 drops lavender
2 drops peppermint

Tenderly blend your bearer oil and
fundamental oils.
Rub enough blend into the scalp to cover.
Leave on for any event for 15 minutes.
Wash out with a delicate cleanser.

Diy Deep Moisturizing Dry Scalp Treatments #2

4 drops tea tree
2 drops lavender
1 drop geranium
1 drop patchouli

Tenderly blend your bearer oil and fundamental oils.
Rub enough blend into the scalp to cover.
Leave on for any event for 15 minutes.
Wash out with a delicate cleanser.

Lemongrass Oil

Lemongrass oil
Shampoo/Conditioner

Lemongrass oil for dandruff is best when utilized every day. Blend a couple of drops into your cleanser or conditioner every day, and ensure it's rubbed into your scalp.

Thyme Essential Oil

2 drops Thyme Essential Oil
5 drops Lavender Essential Oil
2 tbsp Virgin Olive Oil

Rub the mix into the scalp and allow it to
remain for 20 minutes.
Cleanse it out.

Cedarwood Essential Oil

2-3 drops Cedarwood Essential Oil
2 tbsp Coconut Oil
5 drop Cedarwood Essential Oil
1 tbsp Shampoo

Rub your scalp with it, smoothing it through
your hair.
Clean your hair with it.

Tea Tree Oil for Hair Growth and Itchy Scalp

296-591 drops Olive Oil
5 drops Tea Tree Essential Oil
2 tbsp Aloe Vera Gel

Vitamin A present in aloe vera produces healthy sebum, a slick substance discharged by the scalp, which shields hair and scalp from getting out and breaking dry.
Also, Vitamin A battles free radicals that burden your hair.
Nutrient B12 in aloe vera is significant for a sound scalp. Along these lines, it quiets the bothersome scalp. It averts dandruff and disposes of the follicles' trash and empowers the development of new hair.

Tea Tree Oil and Coconut Oil

1-2 tbsp Coconut Oil
5-8 drops Tea Tree Oil

Mix the tea tree oil with the coconut oil.
Presently utilizing your fingers, rub your
scalp with this oil blend.
Concentrate on the dry and flaky scalp fixes,
however, rub the majority of your scalp
Allow it to remain for 30 minutes or
medium-term.
Cleanse it with a cleanser and conditioner.
Rehash 2-3 times each week.

Tea Tree Oil + Shampoo

2 drops Tea Tree Oil
1 oz Shampoo

Restore the bottle of shampoo top and
shake vivaciously before utilizing.
Use it as a shampoo regularly.
This cure dispenses with any parasitic and
bacterial contamination on the scalp that
causes flaky and itchy skin.
Some people should consume tea tree oil.
An individual ought to apply a drop of the oil
to the skin within the wrist to test for any
unfavorable responses.

DIY Natural Hair Moisturizer

2 tbsp of Coconut Oil
1 tbsp of Bio Active Manuka Honey (or any raw honey will work)
1-2 drops of Orange Essential Oil

Start by blending sugar and coconut oil. The coconut oil is generally strong in structure yet leaving it warm for a couple of days will make it genuinely fluid.
Then, add 1 to 2 drops of orange essential oil. I picked orange since I cherish the mixed fragrance of these three fixings together yet you can pick any essential oil of your inclination.
Heat the blend in the microwave for 5 seconds and mix all together.
Before applying, ensure that the blend isn't excessively hot.
At that point, turn your hair over, applying the blend to the center part of the hair up to the finishes.
Gather the hair and clasp in over the head and leave for around 30 minutes.
Wash with warm water.
Apply cleanser and conditioner like the standard thing.

DIY Natural Hair Moisturizer

2 tbsp of Coconut Oil
1 tbsp of Honey
1-2 drops of Orange Essential Oil

Begin by combining the coconut oil with the honey. If coconut oil is solid, allow it to warm up to liquify a bit.
Add a drop or two of orange essential oil. The orange is a personal preference based on my fave scents.
Heat up the mix in the microwave for 5 seconds, and then stir thoroughly.
Check to make sure it is cool enough to touch.
If so, flip your hair upside down and apply the moisturizer to the ends and middle portion of your hair.
Clip it on top of your head and leave in for 25 minutes.
Rinse with warm water and shampoo & condition as usual.

Diy Hair Conditioner

20g Aloe Juice
5g Glycerin
5g BTMS
3g (60 drops) Argan Oil
2g (40 drops) Jojoba Oil
3.5g Natural Preservative like Leucidal (or 1g Rokonsol)
2.5g Wheat Protein
.5g D-panthenol
1g (20 drops) Essential Oils (I used lavender EO)

Weigh out water, aloe juice, and glycerin and combine.
Warmth the blend in a twofold heater.
While waiting, weigh out the oils and BTMS and consolidate.
Put in a twofold heater embedded.
Heat the oils in the twofold evaporator.
Blend continually until the BTMS liquefies and is completely consolidated into the oils.
Expel from warmth.
Combine the boiling water-solvent fixings and the hot oils.
If you see that the blend isolates, this is because of the distinction in temperature.
This can be easily fixed by mixing over warmth in the twofold evaporator embed until it is emulsified.

When the blend is cool enough, you can include different fixings that are heat-touchy, for example, the additives, wheat protein, panthenol, and essential oils. If you are utilizing an additive like Rokonsol that requires a pH of under 5 to be successful, you should include a couple of drops of lactic acid to cut the pH down first.
Put the blend in a jug.
Try not to cover with the top until the blend arrives at room temperature.
This is with the goal that the water does not gather over the conditioner.
Use inside 3 months.

Carrot Seed Conditioner

¼ cup Coconut Oil
¼ cup thick Unflavored Unsweetened
Yogurt
¼ cup Aloe Vera Gel
7 drops Carrot Seed Essential Oil
9 drops Geranium Essential Oil
High speed blender
Mason jar

Combine 1/4 cup of coconut oil, 1/4 cup of
aloe vera gel, and 1/4 cup of thick unflavored
and unsweetened yogurt.
At that point, include the basic oils.
Blend until you get a white blend with a
velvety consistency.
Transfer the blend into an artisan container
or a container that has a water/air proof
cover.
Put in the fridge.
Use 1 tbsp of the blend when you go to the
shower and apply it along the length of your
hair.
Leave for 2 minutes before flushing off with
lukewarm water.
Alternatively, you can likewise utilize this as
a molding hair veil on dry hair yet make a
point to leave it for 40 minutes before

flushing and washing off with a cleanser.

DIY Essential Oil Hair Spray

7 drops Rosemary
10 drops Lavender
3 drops Thyme
3 drops Cedarwood
1 tbsp Witch Hazel
½ cup Distilled Water
4 oz Glass Spray Bottle

To start with, combine all the essential oils
with witch hazel and stir well.
Now take the distilled water or filtered water
and pour it into the glass spray bottle.
Add the prepared solution to this spray
bottle and shake well to combine them.
Keep it in a dry and cool place.

Tea Tree and Apricot Oil Shampoo

240 mL Distilled Water
80 mL Liquid Castile Soap
10 drops Tea Tree Oil
5 mL Apricot Oil

To make tea tree and apricot oil shampoo,
add all the oils onto castile soap and distilled
water altogether.

DIY Natural Shampoo For Curly Hair

2 tbsp of Aloe Vera Gel
½ a cup of Distilled Water.
1 tbsp of Almond Oil.
5 to 8 drops of either Bergamot, Lemon, Orange, Ylang Ylang, Lavender or Frankincense oil.

Essentially blend the water with aloe vera gel and mix well.
At that point include the basic oils while blending to guarantee that they round out the remainder of the blend.
When this is done, you can store the cleaner in a spotless glass or plastic compartment and refrigerate it.
It's ideal to utilize the cleanser on clammy hair.

Natural Blue Shampoo

¼ cup Makes 3 Organics Lavender Orange
Castile Liquid Soap
¼ cup Canned Coconut Milk
½ tbsp of Baking Soda
½ tsp Avocado Oil
5 drops Rosemary Essential Oil
10 drops of Moroccan Blue Chamomile
Essential Oil
10 drops of your choice of Essential Oils that
fit your needs!
Optional Sage or Honey

Add Liquid Soap to the blending bowl and
race in the support soft drink.
Include coconut Milk and Avocado Oil.
At that point include essential oil.
Blend well with whiskey.
Fill a compartment.
We found that when utilizing a frothing
container, the cleanser foams better in hair.
You can reuse one of your Liquid Soap
compartments from Makes 3 Organics, or
get one on the web! I chose to store our
completed item in the ice chest so it would
last longer,
as it may on the off chance that you make it
in little bunches and wash your hair day by
day, cool stockpiling may not be vital.

Your Own EO Blends

Your Own EO Blends

Your Own EO Blends

Book Ordering

To order your copy / copies of
Essential Oils for Dandruff

please visit: **EOrecipes.net**

You can also check out other titles available.

Bulk Pricing and
Affiliate Programs Available

www.ingramcontent.com/pod-product-compliance
Lightning Source LLC
Chambersburg PA
CBHW051416250726
48655CB00003B/1074